The Lost Book of Herbal Remedies.

Unlocking the Healing Power of Plants

"For every disease known to mankind, there is a plant somewhere in the world that holds the cure."

The Herbs are for the healing of the nations. Certified and licensed Herbalist.

FOR PARENTS, HEALTH WORKERS, STUDENTS AND TRADITIONAL DOCTORS

Please take your time reading this instruction manual and absorb its contents fully.

Benson Wilson

Copyright@2024

For more information and support contact:
herbalifenaturescure@gmail.com

All rights reserved @Copyright 2024.

Without the express, explicit permission of the author and/or publisher, no part of this book may be reproduced, transmitted, or copied in any form whatsoever.

Neither the book's publisher nor the author will be held liable for any losses or injuries, financial or otherwise, that may occur as a direct or indirect result of following.

Notice of Legal Effects:

This book is subject to copyright regulations. For your eyes only, if you will. The content may not be modified, copied, sold, used, quoted, or paraphrased in any way without the prior written consent of the author or publisher.

Disclaimer Notice:

Please note that this document is intended for educational and informational purposes only. Every effort has been made to ensure the information is as accurate, current, reliable, and comprehensive as possible. However, the content in this book is derived from various natural herbal sources. If you do not fully understand any of the strategies mentioned, please consult us via email for further clarification before using them.

By using this information, whether or not it contains errors or inaccuracies, you acknowledge that the author is not liable for any direct or indirect damages resulting from your reliance on the content provided.

ISBN: 978-1-300-94570-3

Author: BENSON WILSON

Book Title: The Lost Book of Herbal Remedies: Unlocking the Healing Power of Plants

For more information and support contact:
herbalifenaturescure@gmail.com

Acknowledgment

Thank you from the bottom of my heart to everyone who has helped make **The Lost Book of Herbal Remedies:** Unlocking the Healing Power of Plants. Devotion to the restorative power of nature, together with years of study and personal discovery, has culminated in this book. Everyone who had faith in the power of natural healing and pushed me to investigate herbal therapies has my undying gratitude.

To the traditional healers and herbalists whose insights formed the bedrock of this work, I offer my deepest gratitude. The foundation for many of the cures presented here may be found in their time-honored practices for treating obesity, cancer, fever, and other diseases.

Our deepest gratitude goes out to those who have contributed wisdom on the many facets of human health, especially as it pertains to men's innate sexual drive, women's natural lubrication, and men's strong libido. By bringing together contemporary research and traditional traditions, your contributions have made this book an all-inclusive resource for holistic health.

Last but not least, **The Lost Book of Herbal Remedies** is for those readers who are looking to build a stronger bond between their well-being and the natural world. With any luck, this book will provide you the tools you need to live a full, balanced life by embracing the restorative power of nature.

Incredibly grateful to everyone who has played a role in our adventure. We may keep on healing and thriving by utilizing the natural cures that are all around us if we work together.

For more information and support contact:
herbalifenaturescure@gmail.com

TABLE OF CONTENTS

CHAPTER ONE 8

   BOOST YOUR PASSION: TRIED-AND-TRUE METHODS FOR INCREASING A MAN'S NATURAL SEXUAL DESIRE 8

      Bitter kola, Alligator pepper, Coconut water 8

CHAPTER TWO 10

   UNLOCK ENHANCED PASSION: UNDERSTANDING AND EMBRACING HIGH LIBIDO AND NATURAL LUBRICATION IN WOMEN 10

      GORANTULA REMEDY 10

CHAPTER THREE 12

   Orange leaves Remedies 12

Chapter four 14

   Coconut leaves Remedies 14

Chapter Five 16

   Pineapple peels Remedies 16

Chapter Six 18

   Fever Remedy 18

      Pawpaw (Papaya) leaves 18

Chapter Seven 20

   Plantain Peels Remedies 20

Chapter Eight 22

   Restore Lost Menstruation and Clear Vaginal Infections 22

Chapter Nine 24

   Water Melon Seeds Remedies 24

Chapter Ten 26

   Relief for Waist Pain 26

      Pineapple leaves and Ginger Remedy 26

For more information and support contact:
herbalifenaturescure@gmail.com

Chapter Eleven 28

   Siam Weed (Acheampong, Awolowo leaves, Akintola) Remedies .. 28

Chapter Twelve 30

   Solution for Battling Depression, Sleeplessness, and Anxiety 30

      Powdered Nutmeg 30

Chapter Thirteen 32

   TUBERCULOSIS CURE 32

Chapter Fourteen 34

   Mango tree Remedies 34

Chapter Fifteen 36

   Cock's comb plant Remedies 36

Chapter Sixteen 38

   Garden eggs leaves Remedies 38

Chapter Seventeen 40

   SEVERE CONSTIPATION 40

      Cucumber and Pineapple Remedy 40

Chapter Eighteen 42

   Irregular or Missing Menstruation Solution 42

      Pawpaw/Papaya Remedy 42

Chapter Nineteen 44

   Touch-me-not" plant Remedies 44

Chapter Twenty 46

   Hepatitis B Remedy 46

      Gale of the wind Leave 46

Chapter Twenty-One 48

   Revitalize Your Sexual Health 48

For more information and support contact:
herbalifenaturescure@gmail.com

Cinnamon, Ginger, and Cloves 48

Chapter Twenty-Two 50

Groundnut shell Remedies 50

Chapter Twenty-Three 52

Natural Remedies for Soothing Itching in the Private Area and Thighs 52

Senna alata Leaves 52

Chapter Twenty-Four 54

Dandelion Leaves Remedy 54

For more information and support contact:
herbalifenaturescure@gmail.com

Preface

The Lost Book of Herbal Remedies: Unlocking the Healing Power of Plants" is a voyage into the realm of natural medicine, based on centuries of knowledge passed down through generations. This book is intended to reconnect us with the healing power of the plants around us—remedies that have long been overlooked in the contemporary world.

This guide covers a wide range of health concerns, including rheumatism, skin irritation, depression, diabetes, hepatitis, epilepsy, and sleep difficulties, among many others, and provides easy and efficient techniques to manage them organically. Each treatment comes with practical instructions, making it accessible to everyone looking for alternative remedies to their health problems.

It is my aim that this book will serve as both a resource and an inspiration, encouraging you to embrace nature's healing powers.

Nature heals.

Warm regards.

For more information and support contact:
herbalifenaturescure@gmail.com

CHAPTER ONE

BOOST YOUR PASSION: TRIED-AND-TRUE METHODS FOR INCREASING A MAN'S NATURAL SEXUAL DESIRE

BITTER KOLA, ALLIGATOR PEPPER, COCONUT WATER

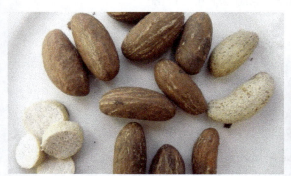
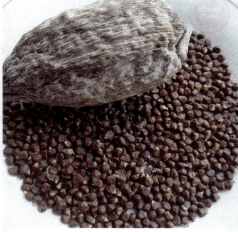
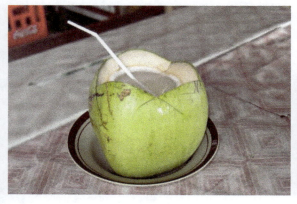
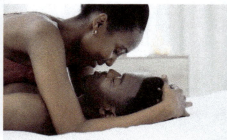

Gentlemen, if you find yourself struggling with endurance during intimate moments, there's no need to worry. Here's a natural remedy that may help boost your stamina.

Illustration

- ❖ Grate six bitter kola nuts into fine shavings.

- ❖ Grind alligator pepper into a smooth, fine powder.

- ❖ Combine the grated bitter kola with the powdered alligator pepper.

- ❖ Add coconut water to the mixture and let it sit for 12 hours to allow the ingredients to blend.

- ❖ Consume this mixture 30 minutes before your intimate moment for potential increased endurance.

This is a natural solution that taps into the wisdom of traditional healing.

Nature's Cure.

For more information and support contact:
herbalifenaturescure@gmail.com

CHAPTER TWO

UNLOCK ENHANCED PASSION: UNDERSTANDING AND EMBRACING HIGH LIBIDO AND NATURAL LUBRICATION IN WOMEN

GORANTULA REMEDY

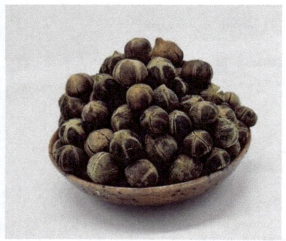

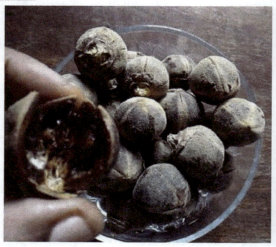

For more information and support contact:
herbalifenaturescure@gmail.com

Gorantula works naturally to enhance a woman's sexual arousal and promote healthy, natural lubrication.

Illustration:

- ❖ Offer her three Gorantula fruits each day for her to enjoy the sweet nectar.

- ❖ This daily intake can boost her natural hydration, elevate her libido, and help reduce vaginal infections.

Nature, through Gorantula, offers a simple yet powerful remedy to enhance her well-being and intimacy.

Nature's Cure.

For more information and support contact:
herbalifenaturescure@gmail.com

CHAPTER THREE
ORANGE LEAVES REMEDIES

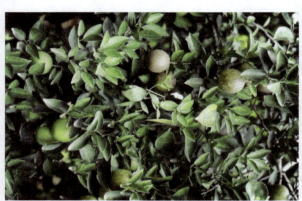
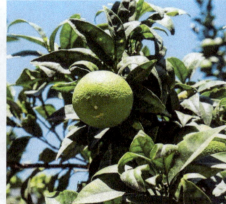
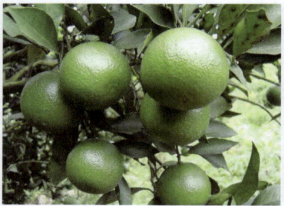
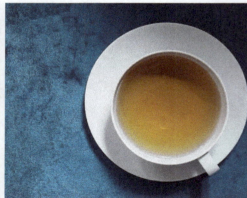

Orange leaves possess potent medicinal properties and can be used to address a variety of health concerns, including:

- Insomnia or difficulty sleeping
- Erectile dysfunction
- Malaria
- Migraines
- Anxiety
- High cholesterol
- Weak immune system
- Menstrual cramps

Illustration:

- ❖ To prepare, boil either fresh or dried orange leaves in water.

- ❖ Drink a teacup of this infusion twice daily for optimal results.

Nature holds the power to restore health and well-being.

Nature's Cure.

For more information and support contact:
herbalifenaturescure@gmail.com

CHAPTER FOUR
COCONUT LEAVES REMEDIES

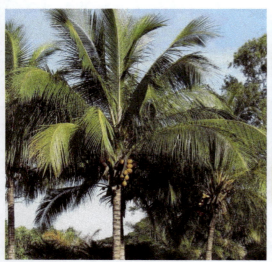
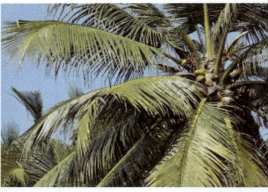
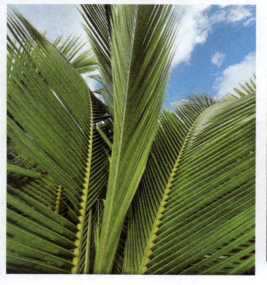
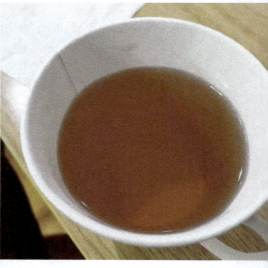

Benefits of Coconut Leaves

Coconut leaves are effective in treating various health issues, including:

- Low sperm count
- Kidney dysfunction
- Obesity
- Diabetes
- Stomach ulcers
- Gonorrhea
- Asthma
- Cough
- High cholesterol

Preparation:

- Measure two tablespoons of dried, powdered coconut leaves and place them into a teacup.

Brewing:

- Pour hot water over the powdered leaves.

Dosage:

- Drink this mixture twice daily.

Nature provides remedies for improved health.

For more information and support contact:
herbalifenaturescure@gmail.com

CHAPTER FIVE

PINEAPPLE PEELS REMEDIES

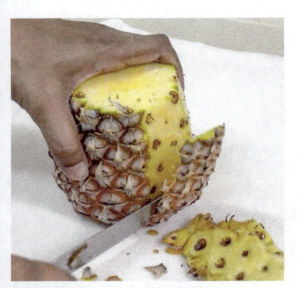
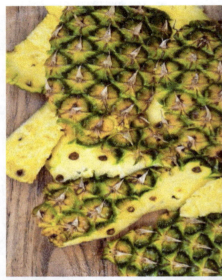
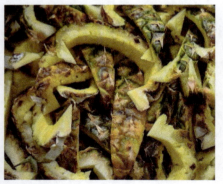
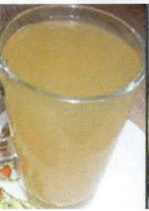
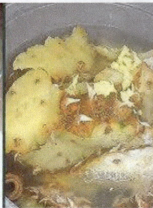

Benefits of Pineapple Peels

Pineapple peels are beneficial in treating a variety of health issues, including:

- Typhoid fever
- Glaucoma
- Arthritis and joint pain
- High cholesterol
- Cold, catarrh, and cough
- Low immunity
- Female infertility

Preparation:

- ❖ Boil the pineapple peels in water for 15 minutes.

Dosage:

- ❖ After boiling, strain the mixture and drink a teacup of the infusion twice daily.

Trust in nature's ability to provide remedies for your health.

For more information and support contact:
herbalifenaturescure@gmail.com

CHAPTER SIX

FEVER REMEDY

PAWPAW (PAPAYA) LEAVES

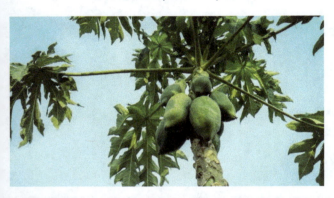
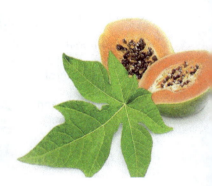
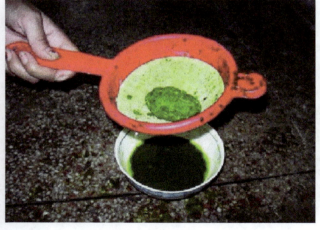
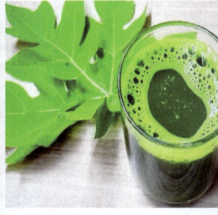

For more information and support contact:
herbalifenaturescure@gmail.com

Quick Remedy for Fever

This simple remedy utilizes the healing properties of pawpaw (papaya) leaves to help reduce fever.

Preparation:

- ❖ Obtain fresh pawpaw leaves.
- ❖ Extraction:
- ❖ Crush the leaves to extract the juice.

Dosage:

- ❖ Drink 2 tablespoons of the juice three times a day for three days.

You will start to feel better soon. Trust in nature's ability to provide effective remedies for your health.

For more information and support contact:
herbalifenaturescure@gmail.com

CHAPTER SEVEN
PLANTAIN PEELS REMEDIES

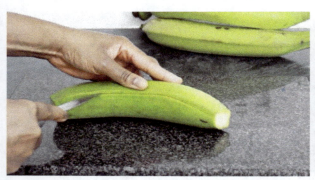
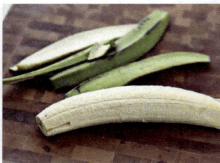
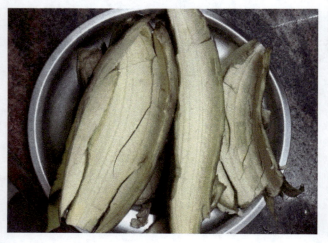
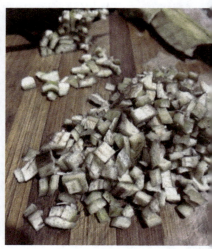

For more information and support contact:
herbalifenaturescure@gmail.com

Uses of Plantain Peels

Plantain peels are beneficial for treating various health issues, including:

- Stomach ulcers
- Acid reflux
- Low sperm count
- Wounds
- Gout
- High prolactin levels
- Kidney stones
- Allergic reactions
- High blood pressure

Preparation:

- ❖ Cut the plantain peels into small pieces.

Cooking:

- ❖ Boil the pieces in water for 15 to 20 minutes.

Dosage:

- ❖ Drink a teacup of the infusion twice daily.

Using plantain peels can help alleviate these conditions effectively.

Nature heals.

For more information and support contact:
herbalifenaturescure@gmail.com

CHAPTER EIGHT

RESTORE LOST MENSTRUATION AND CLEAR VAGINAL INFECTIONS

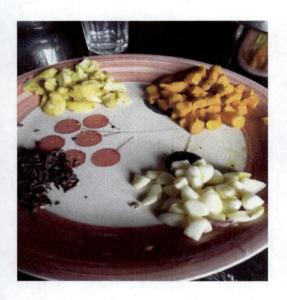
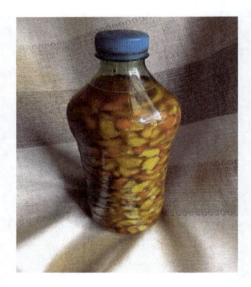
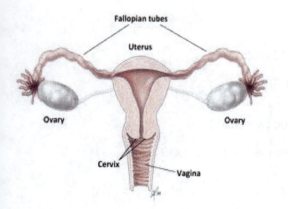
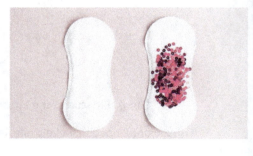

For more information and support contact:
herbalifenaturescure@gmail.com

Restoring Your Menstrual Cycle and Eliminating Vaginal Infections

You can restore your menstrual cycle and eliminate vaginal infections using the following natural ingredients:

❈ Garlic

❈ Turmeric

❈ Cloves

❈ Ginger

Preparation:

- ❖ Peel the outer skin off each ingredient.

Chopping:

- ❖ Cut all the ingredients into small pieces.

Infusion:

- ❖ Place the chopped ingredients in a clean container.

Soaking:

- ❖ Add water to the container and let the mixture sit for 3 days.

Dosage:

- ❖ Drink a teacup of the infusion in the morning and evening.

This natural remedy can help restore your menstrual cycle and reduce vaginal infections.

Nature heals.

For more information and support contact:
herbalifenaturescure@gmail.com

CHAPTER NINE

WATER MELON SEEDS REMEDIES

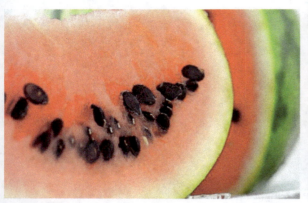
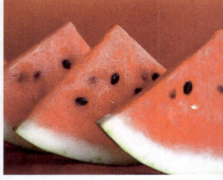
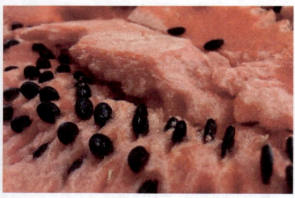
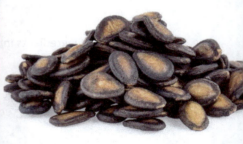

Watermelon Seeds: Benefits for Your Health

Watermelon seeds offer several health benefits, including:

- Enhancing memory power
- Preventing osteoporosis
- Strengthening the immune system
- Preventing hypertension
- Treating erectile dysfunction
- Supporting heart health
- Managing diabetes
- Addressing kidney infections

Illustration:

To gain these benefits, simply chew the seeds along with the fruit.

Nature heals.

For more information and support contact:
herbalifenaturescure@gmail.com

CHAPTER TEN

RELIEF FOR WAIST PAIN

PINEAPPLE LEAVES AND GINGER REMEDY

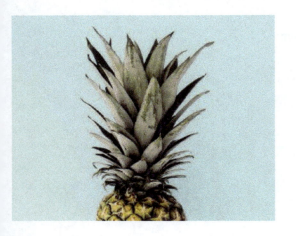
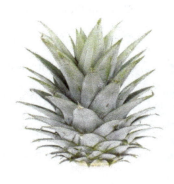
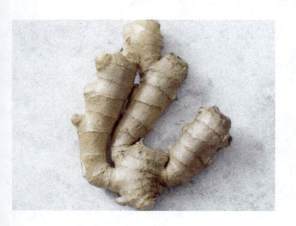
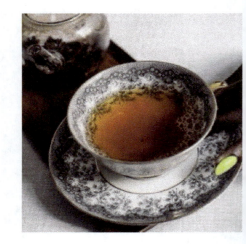

For more information and support contact:
herbalifenaturescure@gmail.com

Relief for Waist Pain

Illustration:

- ❖ Gather pineapple leaves and cut them into small pieces.

- ❖ Add a small amount of ginger to the leaves.

- ❖ Boil the mixture in water.

- ❖ Drink a cup of this infusion twice daily.

This remedy will help relieve your waist pain.

Nature heals.

For more information and support contact:
herbalifenaturescure@gmail.com

CHAPTER ELEVEN

SIAM WEED (ACHEAMPONG, AWOLOWO LEAVES, AKINTOLA) REMEDIES

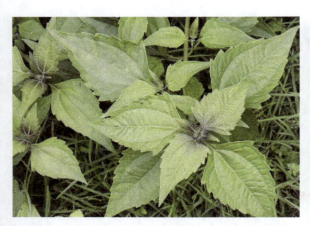
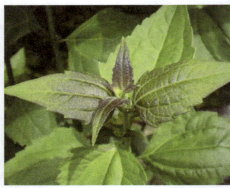
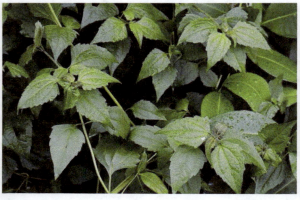
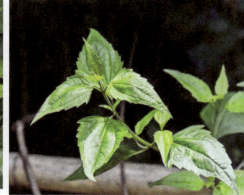

For more information and support contact:
herbalifenaturescure@gmail.com

Siam Weed (Acheampong, Awolowo Leaves, Akintola)

Siam weed is effective in treating:

- Ovarian cysts
- Wounds
- Cervical cancer
- Diabetes
- Hypertension
- Waist pain
- Gout
- Stomach ulcers

Illustration:

- ❖ To prepare the remedy, boil a handful of fresh or dried Siam weed leaves in water.

- ❖ Strain the mixture and drink a teacup of the infusion twice daily.

Nature heals.

CHAPTER TWELVE

SOLUTION FOR BATTLING DEPRESSION, SLEEPLESSNESS, AND ANXIETY

POWDERED NUTMEG

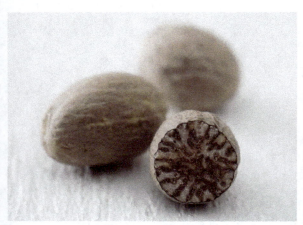
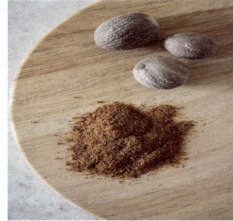
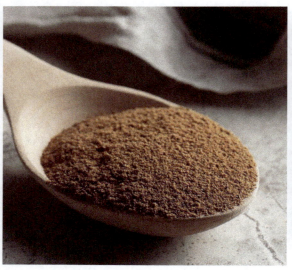
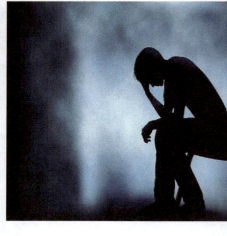

For more information and support contact:
herbalifenaturescure@gmail.com

Relief from Depression, Sleeplessness, and Anxiety

If you are struggling with depression, sleeplessness, or anxiety, there's no need to worry.

Illustration:

- Take a teaspoon of powdered nutmeg.

- Mix it into a glass of hot water.

- Drink this mixture once daily to start feeling better.

Nature heals.

For more information and support contact:
herbalifenaturescure@gmail.com

CHAPTER THIRTEEN
TUBERCULOSIS CURE

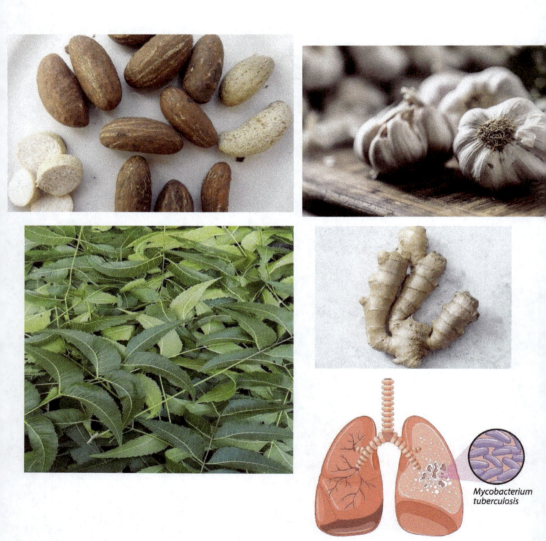

Top Herbs for Treating Tuberculosis

Here are some effective herbs that can help in the treatment of tuberculosis:

Herbs:

🌿 Bitter kola

🌿 Neem tree

🌿 Asthma herb

🌿 Ginger

🌿 Garlic

Illustration:

- ❖ Boil either the Neem tree or Asthma herb in water for 15-20 minutes.

- ❖ Ensure to grate the bitter kola, garlic, and ginger before using them with Neem tree or Asthma for better efficacy.

- ❖ Consume a teacup of the infusion twice daily.

Nature heals.

For more information and support contact:
herbalifenaturescure@gmail.com

CHAPTER FOURTEEN
MANGO TREE REMEDIES

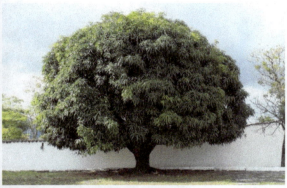
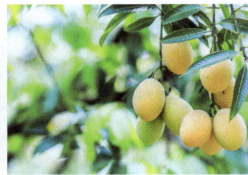
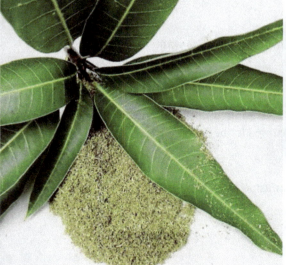
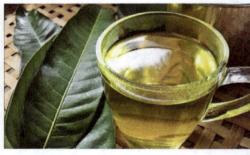

For more information and support contact:
herbalifenaturescure@gmail.com

Mango Tree: Effective Remedies for Various Health Issues

The mango tree offers several health benefits and is effective in treating the following conditions:

Conditions Treated:

🌿 Diabetes

🌿 High blood pressure

🌿 Gallstones

🌿 Kidney stones

🌿 Syphilis

🌿 Malaria

🌿 High cholesterol

🌿 Liver dysfunction

🌿 Anemia

Illustration:

- ❖ Boil two tablespoons of dried, powdered leaves or stem bark in water.

- ❖ Drink this infusion twice daily.

Nature heals.

For more information and support contact:
herbalifenaturescure@gmail.com

CHAPTER FIFTEEN
COCK'S COMB PLANT REMEDIES

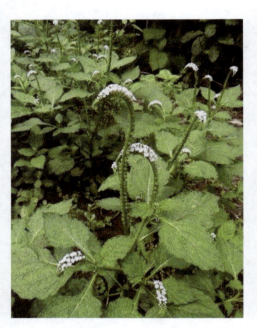
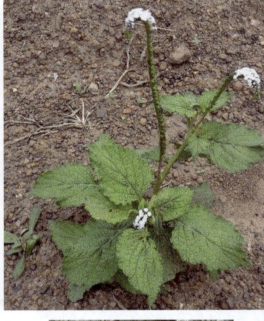
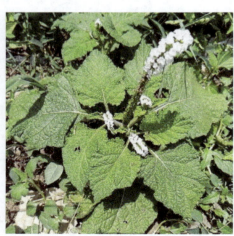
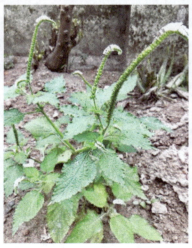

For more information and support contact:
herbalifenaturescure@gmail.com

Cock's Comb Plant: Effective Remedies for Various Health Issues

The cock's comb plant is known for its medicinal properties and is effective in treating the following conditions:

Conditions Treated:

❀ Rheumatism

❀ Sciatica

❀ Gonorrhea

❀ Sore throat

❀ Stomach ulcers

❀ Tumors

❀ Hypertension

❀ Glaucoma

❀ Convulsions

❀ Diabetes

Illustration:

- ❖ Uproot the entire plant.
- ❖ Cut it into pieces.
- ❖ Boil the pieces in water.
- ❖ Drink a teacup of the infusion twice daily for one month.

Nature heals.

For more information and support contact:
herbalifenaturescure@gmail.com

CHAPTER SIXTEEN
GARDEN EGGS LEAVES REMEDIES

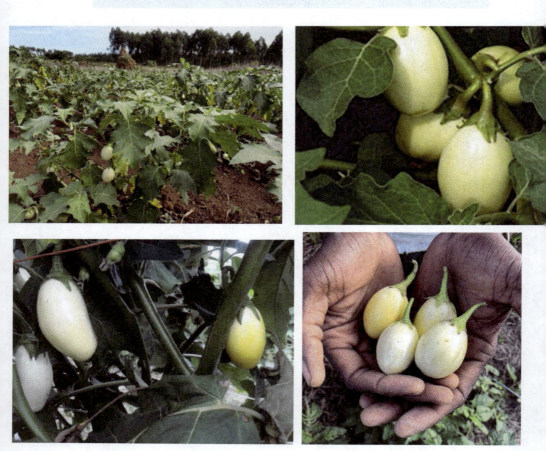

Garden Egg Leaves: Effective Remedies for Various Health Issues

Garden egg leaves possess numerous medicinal properties and can be effective in treating the following conditions:

Conditions Treated:

- Anemia
- Heartburn
- Kidney stones
- Infertility
- Cancer
- Obesity
- Hypertension
- Diabetes
- Stomach ulcers
- General body weakness

Illustration:

- Cut the garden egg leaves into small pieces.
- Boil the pieces in water for 20 minutes.
- Drink a teacup of the infusion twice daily. This remedy works like magic.

Nature heals.

For more information and support contact:
herbalifenaturescure@gmail.com

CHAPTER SEVENTEEN

SEVERE CONSTIPATION

CUCUMBER AND PINEAPPLE REMEDY

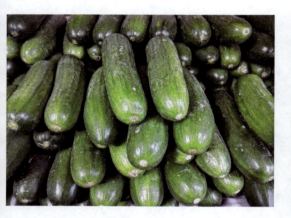
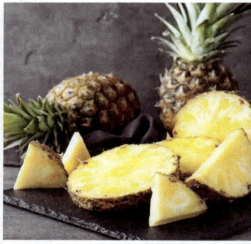
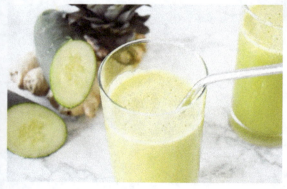
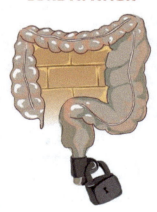

For more information and support contact:
herbalifenaturescure@gmail.com

Relief for Severe Constipation

Illustration:

- ❖ Blend cucumber and pineapple together until smooth.

- ❖ Drink a glass of this mixture for quick relief.

- ❖ This combination not only helps relieve constipation but also detoxifies the colon and eliminates excess waste from the intestines.

For more information and support contact:
herbalifenaturescure@gmail.com

CHAPTER EIGHTEEN

IRREGULAR OR MISSING MENSTRUATION SOLUTION

PAWPAW/PAPAYA REMEDY

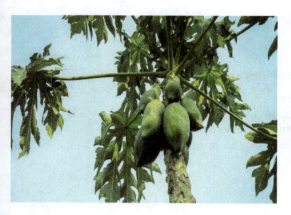
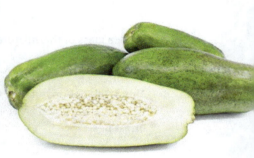
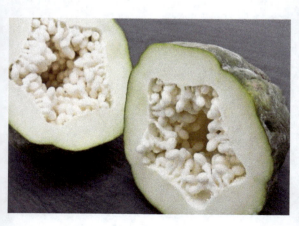
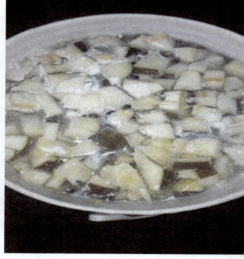

For more information and support contact:
herbalifenaturescure@gmail.com

Addressing Irregular or Missed Menstruation after Contraceptive Use

Illustration:

- ❖ Take unripe pawpaw (papaya) and cut it into small pieces.

- ❖ Boil the pieces in water.

- ❖ Drink four tablespoons of the boiled mixture twice daily for three weeks.

This remedy will help restore your menstrual cycle to normal. Nature heals.

For more information and support contact:
herbalifenaturescure@gmail.com

CHAPTER NINETEEN
TOUCH-ME-NOT" PLANT REMEDIES

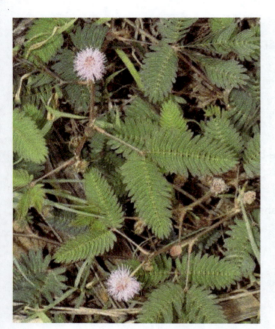
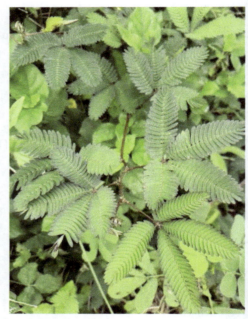
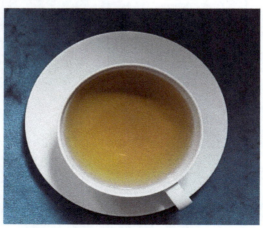

For more information and support contact:
herbalifenaturescure@gmail.com

Benefits of the "Touch-me-not" Plant

The "Touch-me-not" plant is effective in treating the following conditions:

- Epilepsy
- Dementia
- Depression
- Urinary Tract Infection (UTI)
- Anxiety
- Sleep disorders (insomnia)
- Diabetes
- Piles

Illustration:

- ❖ Boil two tablespoons of the dried, powdered whole plant in water for 15 minutes.

- ❖ Drink a teacup of the infusion twice daily.

Nature heals.

For more information and support contact:
herbalifenaturescure@gmail.com

CHAPTER TWENTY

HEPATITIS B REMEDY

GALE OF THE WIND LEAVE

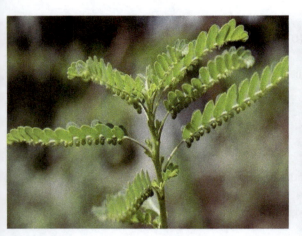
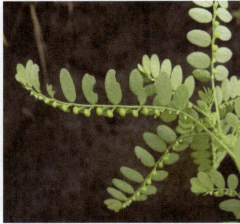
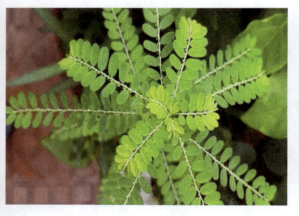
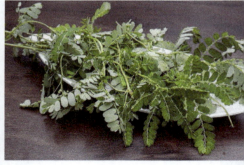

For more information and support contact:
herbalifenaturescure@gmail.com

Hepatitis B Awareness

Hepatitis B Day. Special thanks to this plant for saving countless lives from this dreadful virus.

English: Gale of the Wind

Twi: Bo mma gu wakyi

Yoruba: Ehin olobe

Ga: Ombatoatshi

Illustration:

- ❖ Harvest a handful of the plant.

- ❖ Boil it in water for about 30 to 45 minutes.

- ❖ Take four tablespoons three times daily after meals.

Nature heals.

For more information and support contact:
herbalifenaturescure@gmail.com

CHAPTER TWENTY-ONE

REVITALIZE YOUR SEXUAL HEALTH

CINNAMON, GINGER, AND CLOVES

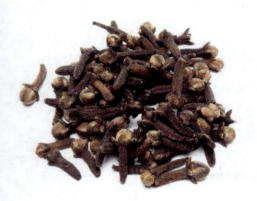
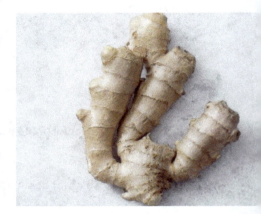
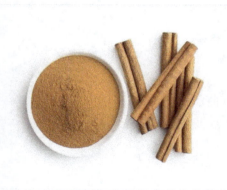
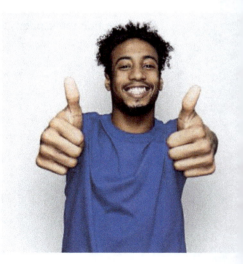

For more information and support contact:
herbalifenaturescure@gmail.com

Restoring Sexual Vitality: A Simple Herbal Remedy

Instructions:

- ❖ Combine cinnamon powder, ginger, and cloves in a pot.

- ❖ Add water and bring the mixture to a boil.

- ❖ Once boiled, let it cool slightly and pour it into a teacup.

- ❖ Drink one teacup of this herbal infusion daily before meals for one week.

This remedy is designed to enhance your sexual health and restore your vitality. Trust in nature's ability to support your well-being!

For more information and support contact:
herbalifenaturescure@gmail.com

CHAPTER TWENTY-TWO
GROUNDNUT SHELL REMEDIES

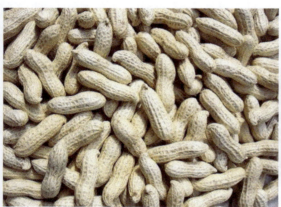
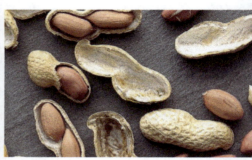
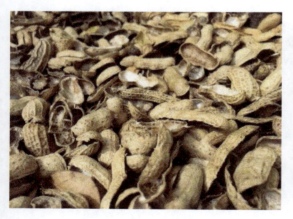
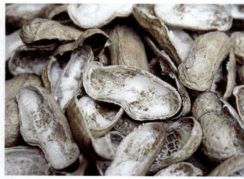

Groundnut Shells: A Natural Remedy for Various Ailments

Benefits: Groundnut shells can help treat:

- Depression
- Diabetes
- Amnesia
- High cholesterol
- Hypertension
- Polycystic Ovary Syndrome (PCOS)
- Stroke
- Poor vision
- Low immunity

Instructions:

- Collect fresh groundnut shells and rinse them.
- Boil the shells in water for 20 minutes.
- Strain the mixture to separate the liquid from the shells.
- Drink a teacup of the infusion twice daily.

Trust in nature's ability to promote healing and improve your health!

For more information and support contact:
herbalifenaturescure@gmail.com

CHAPTER TWENTY-THREE

NATURAL REMEDIES FOR SOOTHING ITCHING IN THE PRIVATE AREA AND THIGHS

SENNA ALATA LEAVES

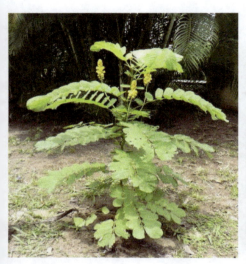
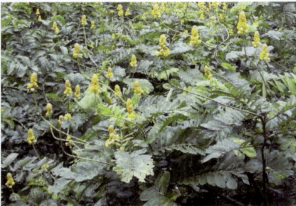
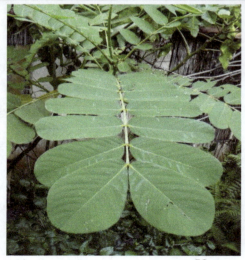

For more information and support contact:
herbalifenaturescure@gmail.com

Herb Remedy for Skin Itching in the Private Area and Thighs

Instructions:

- ❖ Juice Extraction: After taking a bath, press the leaves of the Senna alata plant to extract the juice.

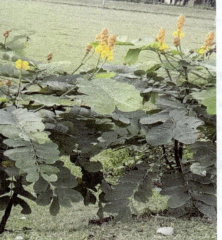

- ❖ Application: Apply the juice directly to the affected areas to relieve itching.

- ❖ Preparation of Herbal Tea: Additionally, boil the leaves in water to create an infusion.

- ❖ Consumption: Drink this infusion twice daily for enhanced relief.

This natural remedy can help soothe irritation and promote healing.

For more information and support contact:
herbalifenaturescure@gmail.com

CHAPTER TWENTY-FOUR

DANDELION LEAVES REMEDY

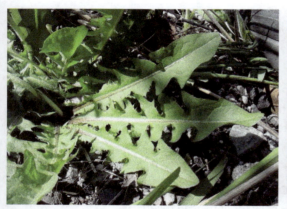
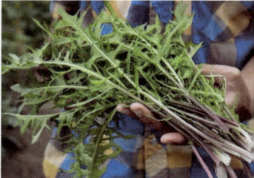
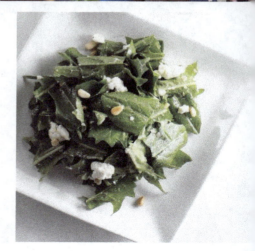

Dandelion: A Natural Remedy for Joint Inflammation

Benefits: Dandelion is an excellent plant for treating:

- ❇ Rheumatism
- ❇ Arthritis

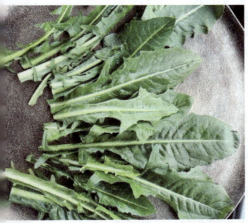

- ❇ Inflamed joints

Instructions:

- ❖ Preparation: Incorporate young dandelion leaves into your salads or meals.
- ❖ Duration: Consume these leaves consistently for 1 to 2 weeks.

With regular use, you will experience complete healing.

Nature heals.

For more information and support contact:
herbalifenaturescure@gmail.com

Thank you all for joining us today to celebrate "The Lost Book of Herbal Remedies." Your presence means a lot!

Dear readers!

I'm truly grateful for your support and interest in "The Lost Book of Herbal Remedies: Unlocking the Healing Power of Plants." Thank you so much! This book is a wonderful guide to tapping into the natural healing powers of plants for a variety of health concerns, such as rheumatism, skin itching, depression, diabetes, hepatitis, epilepsy, sleep disorders, and so much more.

It's wonderful that you're choosing to explore herbal remedies! It shows your dedication to well-being and a holistic approach to health. I'd love for you to share your thoughts by writing a review of the book! Your feedback is super helpful for us to get better and also helps other readers make smart choices about their health!

Also, think about sharing this wonderful resource with students, parents, friends, and medical professionals. The information here can help others appreciate natural healing and encourage a greater understanding of the healing power of plants.

Thanks so much for your purchase! Let's explore the wonderful healing power of nature together!

Best wishes,

For more information and support contact:
herbalifenaturescure@gmail.com